I0441124

Just Tell Me What To Eat

A Guide to Foods and The Benefits of Eating Them

PUBLISHER'S NOTE

The information in this book is as accurate as possible at the time of publication. Please seek the advice of a qualified health professional before attempting to use them. The author, editor, and publisher disclaim all liability (including injuries, damages or losses) resulting from the use of the information in this book. The health information in this book is not intended to be a medical guide for self-treatment.

This book or any portion thereof may not be reproduced or distributed without written permission of the publisher.

RayeQueen

All true foods have nutritional value that our bodies need to perform optimally and to avoid disease. This book is a comprehensive guide to many foods, the benefits of those foods and how it can be used to prevent or treat physical imbalances.

Table of Contents

Table of Contents

ACEROLA CHERRY
Bursting with Vitamin C

Health Properties
- Beta Carotene
- Vitamin C

Eat in Abundance to:
- Protect the heart
- Combat cancer
- Fight fungus
- Lower fever
- Smooth skin
- Support immune system
- Treat diarrhea

EXTRA EXTRA

Look for skin creams that contain acerola to help wipe wrinkles away and clear up other blemishes.

APPLES

High in fiber, vitamins, minerals, and antioxidants

Health Properties
- Fiber
- Vitamin C
- Potassium
- Magnesium
- Pectin
- Antioxidant Quercetin

Eat in Abundance to:
- Protect the heart
- Prevents constipation
- Blocks diarrhea
- Improves lung capacity
- Slows aging process
- Cushions joints

EXTRA EXTRA

Apple cider vinegar is an excellent way to get these nutrients. Make certain you are drinking organic apple cider vinegar with the mother in it.

APRICOTS

Dried apricots have higher amounts of nutrients.

Health Properties
- Beta Carotene
- Iron
- Fiber
- Vitamin C
- B Vitamins
- Carotenoid Lycopene
- Magnesium
- Potassium
- Copper

Eat in Abundance to:
- Combat cancer
- Control blood pressure
- Saves eyesight
- Slows aging process
- Shields against Alzheimer's

EXTRA EXTRA

Avoid dried apricots preserved with sulfites. Avoid all sulfites if you suffer from asthma. Use fresh apricots instead.

ARTICHOKES

Cut off an inch off the top and ½ inch from the tips of the leaves and dispose. These parts are inedible.

Health Properties
- Vitamin C
- Potassium
- Magnesium

Eat in Abundance to:
- Aids digestion
- Lowers cholesterol
- Stabilizes blood sugar
- Protects the heart
- Guards against liver disease

EXTRA EXTRA

Artichokes can cause rashes in some people. It is not very common but not dangerous. If you experience a rash, discontinue eating artichokes.

AVOCADOS

Comes in green, dark purple or almost black, bumpy or smooth.

Health Properties
- Monounsaturated fat
- Potassium
- Fiber
- Vitamin C
- Vitamin E
- Folate
- Glutathione

Eat in Abundance to:
- Lower cholesterol
- Controls blood pressure
- Helps stop strokes
- Battles diabetes
- Combats cancer
- Smoothes skin
- Stimulate hair growth

EXTRA EXTRA
Ripe avocados should be soft enough to give way to gentle pressure.

BANANAS

Probably the cheapest fruit you'll find in your grocery store with only about 100 calories.

Health Properties
- Potassium
- Folate
- Vitamin B6
- Vitamins A
- Vitamins C

Eat in Abundance to:
- Protects your heart
- Controls your blood pressure
- Strengthens bones
- Blocks diarrhea
- Quiets a cough
- Regulates sleep pattern

EXTRA EXTRA
Avoid eating bananas and other foods rich in potassium if you suffer from kidney disease.

BARLEY

Don't expect to get your fiber from drinking barley beer. Most breweries remove the beta-glucan which is where the fiber can be found.

Health Properties
- Potassium
- Phosphorus
- Magnesium
- Iron
- Fiber

Eat in Abundance to:
- Lower cholesterol
- Control blood pressure
- Combat cancer
- Battle diabetes
- Prevent constipation
- Treat stomach disorders
- Treat urinary tract infections

EXTRA EXTRA
If you suffer from Celiac Disease, gluten intolerance or Rheumatoid Arthritis, avoid barley because it contains gluten and lectins.

BEANS

Increase your vitamin C intake to help absorb the type of iron not easily absorbed by the body when consuming beans.

Health Properties
- Protein
- Fiber
- L-Arginine (protein that increases blood flow)

Eat in Abundance to:
- Prevent constipation
- Helps hemorrhoids
- Lowers cholesterol
- Combats cancer
- Prevents sexual function
- Stabilizes blood sugar

EXTRA EXTRA
If you change the water a few times while boiling beans you can greatly reduce the amount of gas they produce.

BEETS

Beets have the highest sugar content of any vegetable.

Health Properties
- Potassium
- Magnesium
- Beta Carotene
- Folate

Eat in Abundance to:
- Combat cancer
- Protect your heart
- Control blood pressure
- Aid weight loss
- Strengthen bones

EXTRA EXTRA
Especially beneficial for women who drink alcohol everyday because of their increased risk of breast cancer. Alcohol disrupts folate absorption.

BLUEBERRIES

Blueberries provide a concentrated source of antioxidants.

Health Properties
- Vitamin C
- Fiber
- Calcium
- Iron
- Antioxidant Anthocyanin

Eat in Abundance to:
- Combats cancer
- Protects your heart
- Stabilizes blood sugar
- Boosts memory
- Fights urinary tract infections
- Prevents constipation

EXTRA EXTRA
Use or freeze blueberries within 5 days

BROCCOLI

Ounce for ounce, broccoli has more than twice as much vitamin C as oranges.

Health Properties
- Vitamin C
- Folate
- Vitamin A
- Potassium
- Calcium
- Phytochemicals
- Carotenoids lutein and zeaxanthin

Eat in Abundance to:
- Strengthen bones
- Saves your eyesight
- Combats prostate cancer
- Battles breast cancer
- Combats colon cancer
- Protects your heart
- Controls blood pressure

EXTRA EXTRA
Do not wash broccoli until you're ready to eat.

BULGUR

Available in coarse, medium, and fine.

Health Properties
- Fiber
- Antioxidants
- Phytoestrogens

Eat in Abundance to:
- Combat digestive, colon, and hormone related cancers
- Protect your heart
- Battle diabetes
- Promote weight loss
- Helps stop strokes

EXTRA EXTRA
Coarse bulgur cooks up like rice.

CABBAGE

Cabbage is a low fat vegetable.

Health Properties
- Anti-cancer enzymes
- Protein
- Fiber
- Vitamin K
- Vitamin C
- Folate
- Manganese
- Vitamin B6

Eat in Abundance to:
- Protect against breast cancer
- Prevent constipation
- Protect your heart
- Promotes weight loss
- Helps hemorrhoids

EXTRA EXTRA
Avoid if you've had stomach surgery or a
peptic ulcer.

CANTALOUPE

Buy cantaloupe that is heavy for its size.

Health Properties
- Potassium
- Fiber
- Folate
- Beta Carotene
- Vitamin C

Eat in Abundance to:
- Saves your eyesight
- Controls blood pressure
- Lowers cholesterol
- Combats cancer
- Supports immune system

EXTRA EXTRA
If your cantaloupe is ripe store it in the refrigerator. If it's hard, store it at room temperature until it's ripe.

CARROTS

Avoid carrots that have root like hairs
growing out of them.

Health Properties
- Fiber
- Beta carotene
- Alpha carotene

Eat in Abundance to:
- Combat breast, and lung cancer
- Protect your eyes
- Saves your eyesight
- Prevents constipation
- Promotes weight loss

EXTRA EXTRA
Beta carotene is most beneficial taken as food.
Studies have determined beta carotene
supplements are ineffective.

CAULIFLOWER

Cauliflower is available year round.

Health Properties
- Vitamin C
- Vitamin K
- Folate
- Fiber

Eat in Abundance to:
- Protects against prostate cancer
- Combats breast cancer
- Strengthens bones
- Banishes bruises
- Guards against heart disease

EXTRA EXTRA
Vitamin K causes blood clotting that could
work against blood thinning medication.
Avoid if you suffer from gout.

CHERRIES

20 tart cherries are at least as effective as other pain-killing medications such as aspirin, ibuprofen and other nonsteroidal anti-inflammatory drugs.

Health Properties
- Flavonoids
- Fiber
- Potassium
- Vitamin A
- Vitamin C
- Antioxidant anthocyanins

Eat in Abundance to:
- Eases arthritis
- Fights gout
- Combats cancer
- Protects your heart
- Ends insomnia
- Shields against Alzheimer's
- Slows aging process

EXTRA EXTRA
Cherries have the highest concentration of melatonin of any fruit.

CHESTNUTS

Very low in fat.

Health Properties
- High quality protein
- Vitamin C
- Complex Carbohydrates

Eat in Abundance to:
- Promotes weight loss
- Protects your heart
- Lowers cholesterol
- Combats cancer
- Controls blood pressure

EXTRA EXTRA
Store nuts in a cool, dry place.

CHILI PEPPERS

A whole pepper provides you with one and a half times the vitamin C or an orange.

Health Properties
- Beta carotene
- Vitamin C
- Capsaicin

Eat in Abundance to:
- Aids digestion
- Soothes a sore throat
- Tames pain
- Combats cancer
- Clears sinuses
- Boosts your immune system

EXTRA EXTRA
Do not eat chili peppers if you suffer from heartburn.

CRANBERRIES

Fresh cranberries are available from October through December.

Health Properties
- Flavonoids
- Vitamin C
- Potassium
- Fiber

Eat in Abundance to:
- Fights urinary tract infections
- Protects your heart
- Combats cancer
- Guards against ulcers
- Kills bacteria

EXTRA EXTRA
You can refrigerate them for two months and freeze them for a year.

CURRANTS

The healthiest currant is the black currant, which is loaded with vitamin C, potassium, and ellagic acid, a substance that fights cancer.

Health Properties
- Vitamin C
- Potassium
- Ellagic Acid
- Fiber

Eat in Abundance to:
- Combat lung, liver, skin, esophagus, and colon cancer
- Protect your heart
- Support immune system
- Helps stop strokes
- Aids digestion
- Controls blood pressure

EXTRA EXTRA
Fresh currants are only available from June to August.

FIGS

Pound for pound, figs pack more fiber than
any other fruit or vegetable.

Health Properties
- Polyphenols
- Fiber
- Potassium
- Magnesium

Eat in Abundance to:
- Lowers cholesterol
- Helps stop strokes
- Controls blood pressure
- Promotes weight loss
- Battles diabetes

EXTRA EXTRA

Figs contain histamine that can irritate your
skin. It can also cause high blood pressure,
headaches, and neck pain if you're taking
antidepressants. Also avoid figs if you have
liver problems

FISH

You can find omega-6 in plenty of foods but omega-3's are found mostly in fish and green leafy vegetables.

Health Properties
- Omega-3 fatty acids
- Antioxidants
- Protein
- Vitamin D

Eat in Abundance to:
- Combat cancer
- Protect the heart
- Boost memory
- Eases arthritis

EXTRA EXTRA
Salmon, mackerel, tuna, pacific herring, anchovy, and bluefish are all good sources of omega-3.

FLAX

Do not take more than five tablespoons of flaxseed oil per day.

Health Properties
- Omega-3 fatty acids
- Alpha linolenic acid

Eat in Abundance to:
- Aid digestion
- Ease arthritis pain
- Protect your heart
- Battle diabetes
- Improve brain health
- Boost immune system

EXTRA EXTRA
Do not fry with flaxseed oil because it loses its nutritional value.

GARLIC

Can be dangerous if taking blood-thinning medications.

Health Properties
- Allicin
- Antioxidants
- Vitamin C
- Flavonoids

Eat in Abundance to:
- Lowers cholesterol
- Controls blood pressure
- Boosts immune system
- Kills bacteria
- Combats cancer
- Fights fungus

EXTRA EXTRA
Do not store garlic in plastic bags, sealed containers, or direct sunlight.

GINGER

Pick ginger with thick branches and tight skin.
Do not purchase cracked or shriveled ginger.

Health Properties
- Phytochemicals
- Antioxidants

Eat in Abundance to:
- Stop nausea
- Fight cancer
- Aids digestion
- Eases arthritis pain
- Increase blood flow
- Soothes heartburn

EXTRA EXTRA
Store ginger at room temperature. Avoid if
taking blood thinners or regularly take
NSAIDs.

GRAPEFRUIT

Grapefruit can interfere with absorption of medications. Grapefruit juice can increase risk of kidney stones.

Health Properties
- Potassium
- Inositol
- Vitamin C
- Pectin
- Lycopene
- Potassium

Eat in Abundance to:
- Protects against heart attack
- Helps with weight loss
- Assists in stopping strokes
- Fights lung, breast, and prostate cancer
- Lowers cholesterol

EXTRA EXTRA
Store grapefruit at room temperature for a week or refrigerated for up to six weeks.

GRAPES

Red grapes protect against age-related macular degeneration, the leading cause of vision loss in people over 50.

Health Properties
- Polyphenols
- Fiber
- Potassium
- Calcium
- Manganese
- Iron
- Resveratrol
- Quercetin

Eat in Abundance to:
- Strengthens the heart
- Fights cancer
- Rebuilds eyesight
- Fights kidney stones
- Increases blood flow
- Fight inflammation

EXTRA EXTRA
Store in the refrigerator in a plastic bag for about a week.

GREEN TEA

Steep green tea in hot water rather than boiled water because boiled destroys some of the antioxidants.

Health Properties
- Antioxidants
- B Vitamins
- Vitamin C
- Theanine

Eat in Abundance to:
- Fight cancer
- Strengthen your heart
- Help stop strokes
- Encourage weight loss
- Strengthen bones
- Kill bacteria

EXTRA EXTRA
Drink decaffeinated tea is caffeine gives you the jitters.

GUAVA

Buy guavas that slightly give to gentle pressure.

Health Properties
- Vitamin C
- Potassium
- Lycopene

Eat in Abundance to:
- Controls blood pressure
- Lowers cholesterol
- Fights diabetes
- Fights cancer
- Protect prostate

EXTRA EXTRA
Guavas should be consumed within one or two days of ripening.

HONEY

Used for centuries as a protective barrier over wounds.

Health Properties
- Antioxidant
- Phenols
- Flavonoids
- Vitamin E

Eat in Abundance to:
- Heal wounds
- Aid digestion
- Fight allergies
- Fight fatigue
- Relieves bloating and cramping

EXTRA EXTRA
Use a a skin moisturizer and anti-wrinkle application.

KALE

Highest ORAC Score (oxygen radical absorbance capacity) of any vegetable

Health Properties
- Vitamin C
- Calcium
- Antioxidants
- Beta carotene
- Lutein
- Vitamin K

Eat in Abundance to:
- Strengthen eyesight
- Build healthy bones
- Fight cancer
- Encourage weight loss
- Boosts the immune system

EXTRA EXTRA
Store kale in the refrigerator. Eat within a day or two.

MANGOES

Mangoes make a good meat tenderizer.

Health Properties
- Beta carotene
- Vitamin C
- Vitamin B6
- Vitamin E
- Potassium

Eat in Abundance to:
- Fight cancer
- Enhances memory
- Regulates thyroid
- Helps digestion

EXTRA EXTRA
Mangoes ripen at room temperature.

LEMONS & LIMES

You'll get more juice from a lemon that's at room temperature.

Health Properties
- Vitamin C
- Antioxidants
- Phytochemicals

Eat in Abundance to:
- Fight cancer
- Strengthen your heart
- Control blood pressure
- Combats scurvy

EXTRA EXTRA
Lemons should feel heavy for their size.

MUSHROOMS

Shiitake, maitake, and chanterelle are the most nutritious of all mushrooms.

Health Properties
- Polysaccharides
- Selenium
- Vitamin D

Eat in Abundance to:
- Controls blood pressure
- Fights bacteria
- Lowers cholesterol
- Fights cancer
- Strengthens bones
- Build immune system

EXTRA EXTRA
It's best to buy mushrooms fresh.

OATS

Be careful about buying instant oatmeal. It contains added sugar and salt.

Health Properties
- Beta-glucan
- Protein
- Potassium
- Magnesium
- Phosphorus
- Manganese
- Copper
- Zinc

Eat in Abundance to:
- Lower cholesterol
- Fight cancer
- Fight diabetes
- Prevent constipation
- Reduce risk of stroke
- Promote healthy skin

EXTRA EXTRA
Oats contain gluten. Avoid if you have celiac disease or a gluten sensitivity.

OKRA

The health properties in okra help build up joints and cartilage.

Health Properties
- Potassium
- Vitamin C
- Magnesium
- Folate
- Manganese
- Beta carotene

Eat in Abundance to:
- Builds strong bones
- Strengthens the heart
- Minimizes arthritis
- Controls blood pressure
- Increase blood circulation

EXTRA EXTRA
Recent studies indicate okra might help level blood sugar levels.

OLIVE OIL

Purchase extra virgin olive oil and store at room temperature.

Health Properties
- Monounsaturated fat
- Vitamin E
- Antioxidants

Eat in Abundance to:
- Protect your heart
- Encourage weight loss
- Fight cancer
- Fight arthritis
- Fight diabetes
- Promote smooth skin

EXTRA EXTRA
Use extra virgin olive oil in your skin care routine, to treat wounds, eczema, and psoriasis.

ONIONS

Store onions in a cool, dry place. Store unused portion of onion in refrigerator for up to four days.

Health Properties
- Flavonoid Quercetin
- Sulfur compounds
- Potassium
- Vitamin C
- B Vitamins

Eat in Abundance to:
- Keep heart attacks at bay
- Fight cancer
- Destroy bacteria
- Lower cholesterol
- Fight fungus
- Help stop strokes

EXTRA EXTRA
Cut onion under running water, or place in the refrigerator an hour before slicing to help avoid the tears

ORANGES

Keep oranges at room temperature for a day or two or in the refrigerator for two weeks.

Health Properties
- Vitamin C
- Carotenoids
- Folate
- Fiber
- Potassium

Eat in Abundance to:
- Support immune system
- Fight cancer
- Strengthen your heart
- Strengthen respiratory system

EXTRA EXTRA
Too much vitamin C can cause diarrhea or other stomach problems.

PARSLEY

Eating parsley may reduce your risk of hormone related cancers.

Health Properties
- Vitamin C
- Beta carotene
- Folate
- Iron
- Vitamin K

Eat in Abundance to:
- Strengthen your heart
- Fight cancer
- Build strong bones
- Combat urinary tract infections
- Freshen breath

EXTRA EXTRA
Too much parsley might interact with blood-thinning medications.

PEACHES

Buy organic as peaches are known for being highly treated with pesticides.

Health Properties
- Vitamin A
- Vitamin C
- Phytochemicals

Eat in Abundance to:
- Fight constipation
- Fight cancer
- Help stop strokes
- Boost your immune system
- Helps hemorrhoids

EXTRA EXTRA
When buying canned peaches, purchase ones in its own juice.

PEANUTS

Natural peanut butter should be refrigerated after opening.

Health Properties
- Protein
- Fiber
- Vitamin E
- Niacin
- Manganese
- Folate
- Magnesium
- Potassium

Eat in Abundance to:
- Fight heart disease
- Enhance weight loss
- Fight prostate cancer
- Lower cholesterol
- Fight fatigue

EXTRA EXTRA
Peanuts are one of the most common sources of allergy.

PINEAPPLE

Pineapple has been used to dissolve warts.

Health Properties
- Bromelain
- Vitamin C
- Manganese

Eat in Abundance to:
- Build bones
- Temper cold symptoms
- Aid digestion
- Stop diarrhea

EXTRA EXTRA

Natural cough syrup - 8 ounces of warm pineapple juice and 2 tsp honey.

PRUNES

Also known as dried plum

Health Properties
- Fiber
- Potassium
- Antioxidants

Eat in Abundance to:
- Age slowly
- Prevent constipation
- Lower cholesterol
- Enhance memory
- Encourage weight loss
- Fight heart disease

EXTRA EXTRA
Have the highest ORAC Score (Oxygen Radical Absorbance Capacity

PUMKIN

Men who eat a handful a day ward off prostate problems.

Health Properties
- Beta carotene
- Alpha carotene
- Fiber
- Iron
- Potassium
- Magnesium

Eat in Abundance to:
- Strengthen prostate
- Prolong sexual abilities
- Fight arthritis
- Protect the heart
- Lowers cholesterol

EXTRA EXTRA
Scientists are in the process of confirming pumpkin seed oil may improve the effectiveness of medications used to treat high blood pressure.

QUINOA

One of the healthiest foods you'll find.

Health Properties
- Amino acids
- B Vitamins
- Fiber
- Protein
- Insoluble and soluble fiber

Eat in Abundance to:
- Fight cancer
- Strengthen your heart
- Fight anemia
- Build strong bones
- Help strengthen eyesight

EXTRA EXTRA
Make sure to thoroughly rinse quinoa before cooking.

RICE

All rice starts off brown in color. It should be eaten that way.

Health Properties
- Fiber
- Thiamine

Eat in Abundance to:
- Fight cancer
- Dissolve kidney stones
- Help stop strokes
- Fight diabetes
- Strengthen your heart

EXTRA EXTRA
Brown rice contains extra protein.

SEA VEGETABLES

You can find dried sheets of many sea vegetables at Asian markets and some health food stores.

Health Properties
- Selenium
- Iodine
- Magnesium
- Calcium
- Iron
- Beta carotene
- Antioxidants
- Fiber

Eat in Abundance to:
- Fight cancer
- Fights viruses
- Fights anemia
- Strengthen your heart
- Builds your immune system

EXTRA EXTRA
Nori is loaded with B12.

SPINACH

Large amounts of spinach can block calcium absorption.

Health Properties
- Iron
- Magnesium
- Manganese
- Folate
- Vitamin A
- Vitamin C
- Vitamin K

Eat in Abundance to:
- Protect eyesight
- Boost immune system
- Help stop strokes
- Build strong bones
- Fight cancer
- Strengthen heart

EXTRA EXTRA

Unlike most veggies, iron and beta carotene from spinach are absorbed better when cooked.

SWEET POTATOES

Sweet potatoes and yams are actually two separate vegetables.

Health Properties
- Folate
- Vitamin C
- Beta carotene
- Vitamin B6

Eat in Abundance to:
- Protect eyesight
- Fight cancer
- Boost immune system
- Fight depression
- Strengthen heart

EXTRA EXTRA

Store sweet potatoes and yams out in the open where they will last up to ten days.

STRAWBERRIES

Buy local strawberries. There have been many health scares from frozen ones sent from overseas.

Health Properties
- Vitamin C
- Fiber
- Folate
- Potassium
- Antioxidants

Eat in Abundance to:
- Fight cancer
- Enhance cognition
- Strengthen your heart
- Promotes relaxation

EXTRA EXTRA
Strawberries will keep for about a week in the refrigerator.

TOMATOES

Most people believe tomatoes are vegetables. Most people would be wrong. Tomatoes are fruit.

Health Properties
- Lycopene
- Vitamin C
- Folate
- Potassium

Eat in Abundance to:
- Protects the prostate
- Strengthen the heart
- Fight cancer
- Build the immune system
- Lower cholesterol

EXTRA EXTRA
Store tomatoes in a paper bag, not in the refrigerator.

TURMERIC
Tumeric can aggravate gallstones.

Health Properties
- Curcumin
- Phytochemicals

Eat in Abundance to:
- Reduces inflammation
- Fights arthritis
- Fights cancer
- Protects the liver
- Eases digestion

EXTRA EXTRA
Turmeric has also been known to fight depression.

WALNUTS

Walnuts contain a lot of fat so don't go overboard.

Health Properties
- Polyunsaturated fat
- Alpha Linolenic acid
- Vitamin E
- Ellagic acid

Eat in Abundance to:
- Strengthen the heart
- Lowers cholesterol
- Fight depression
- Fight cancer
- Increase blood flow
- Boosts your memory

EXTRA EXTRA
Store walnuts in a cool dry place for up to three months.

WATER

Health Properties

You can survive over a month without food but only 10 days without water. 75% of our bodies are composed with water. Drink about six full glasses of water daily.

Drink in Abundance to:

- Encourages weight loss
- Fights cancer
- Dissolves kidney stones
- Fights arthritis
- Promotes healthy skin

EXTRA EXTRA

Do not wait until you're thirsty to drink water. There is a good chance you are already dehydrated if you're thirsty.

WATERMELON

Watermelon contains 92% water.

Health Properties
- Vitamin A
- Vitamin C
- Potassium
- Lycopene

Eat in Abundance to:
- Helps stop strokes
- Strengthens the prostate
- Encourages weight loss
- Controls blood pressure
- Lowers cholesterol

EXTRA EXTRA

The juiciest watermelons have a yellow area on it.

YOGURT

Buy yogurt with live active cultures.

Health Properties

- Calcium
- Riboflavin
- Protein
- Vitamin B12
- Potassium
- Active cultures

Eat in Abundance to:

- Lowers cholesterol
- Helps digestion
- Builds immune system
- Builds strong bones
- Protects against ulcers
- Fights yeast

EXTRA EXTRA

Use as a substitute for mayonnaise.

INDEX

INDEX

www.ingramcontent.com/pod-product-compliance
Lightning Source LLC
Chambersburg PA
CBHW071241280526
45788CB00004B/1527